MY FIRST HAIRCUT

BY MARY CAHOE AND
ILLUSTRATED BY NAIRA TANGAMYAN

Gary's
BARBER SHOP

My First Haircut

iUniverse books may be ordered through booksellers or by contacting:

iUniverse
1663 Liberty Drive
Bloomington, IN 47403
www.iuniverse.com
844-349-9409

Because of the dynamic nature of the Internet, any web addresses or links contained in this book may have changed since publication and may no longer be valid. The views expressed in this work are solely those of the author and do not necessarily reflect the views of the publisher, and the publisher hereby disclaims any responsibility for them.

Any people depicted in stock imagery provided by Getty Images are models, and such images are being used for illustrative purposes only. Certain stock imagery © Getty Images.

ISBN: 978-1-6632-2703-4 (sc)
ISBN: 978-1-6632-2704-1 (e)

Library of Congress Control Number: 2021915303

Print information available on the last page.

iUniverse rev. date: 08/12/2021

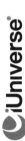
iUniverse®

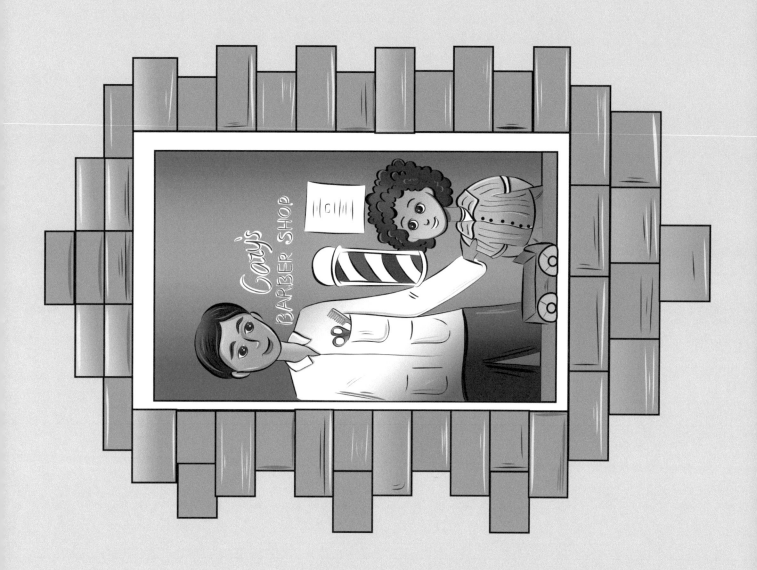

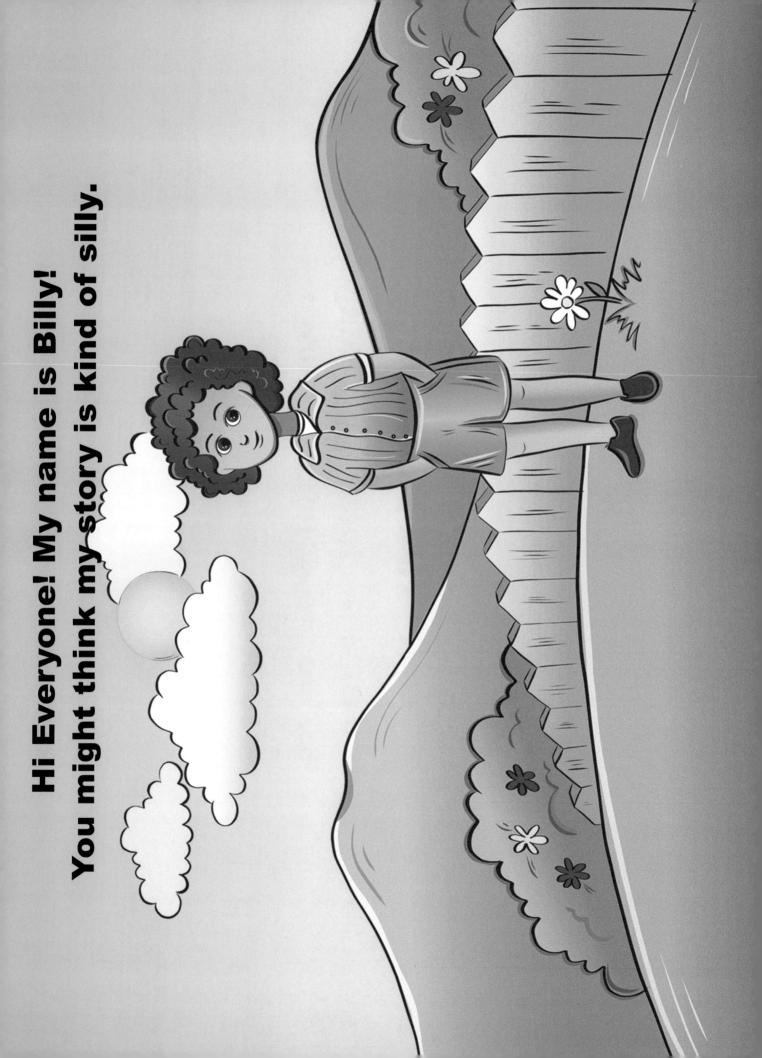

Hi Everyone! My name is Billy!
You might think my story is kind of silly.

Something new happened to me.

It started when my Mom sat down

next to me and said,

"Little Billy we have something to

do. We are going downtown

to do something new."

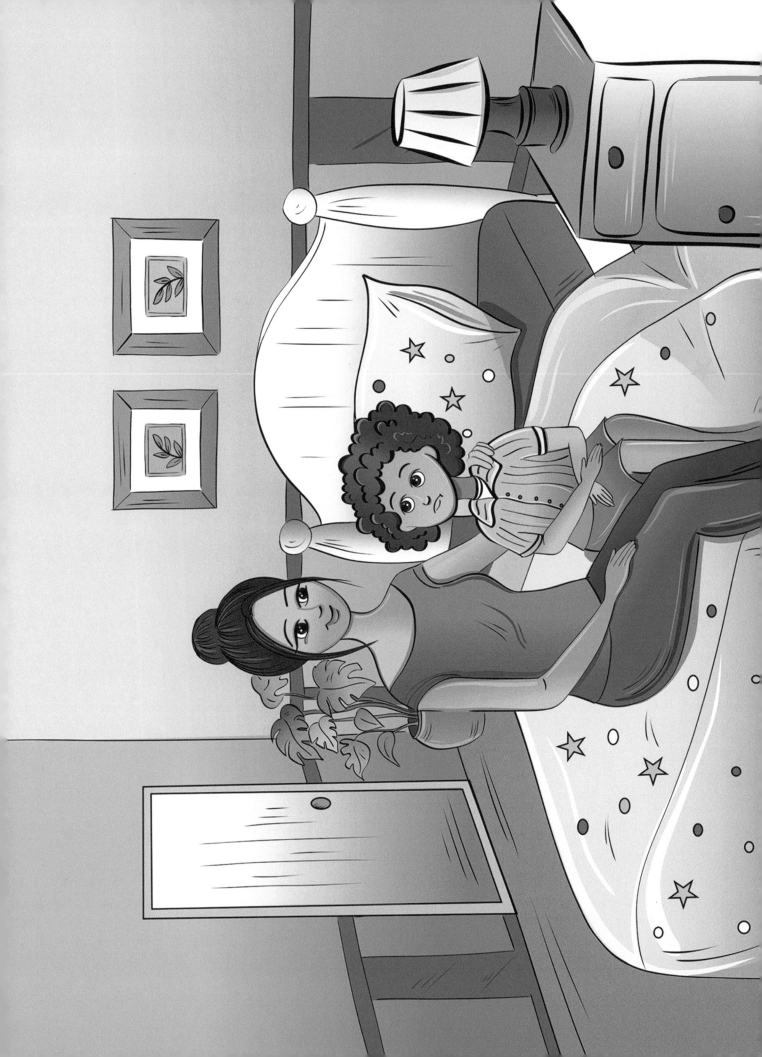

I asked, "What is it Mommy? Is it new shoes?

Is it a new ball? Please tell me the news!

"No, it is something so new you have never done it, and it is time that you do."

"Please Mommy, tell me, I can't hardly wait!"

"You are getting a haircut. It will be great!"

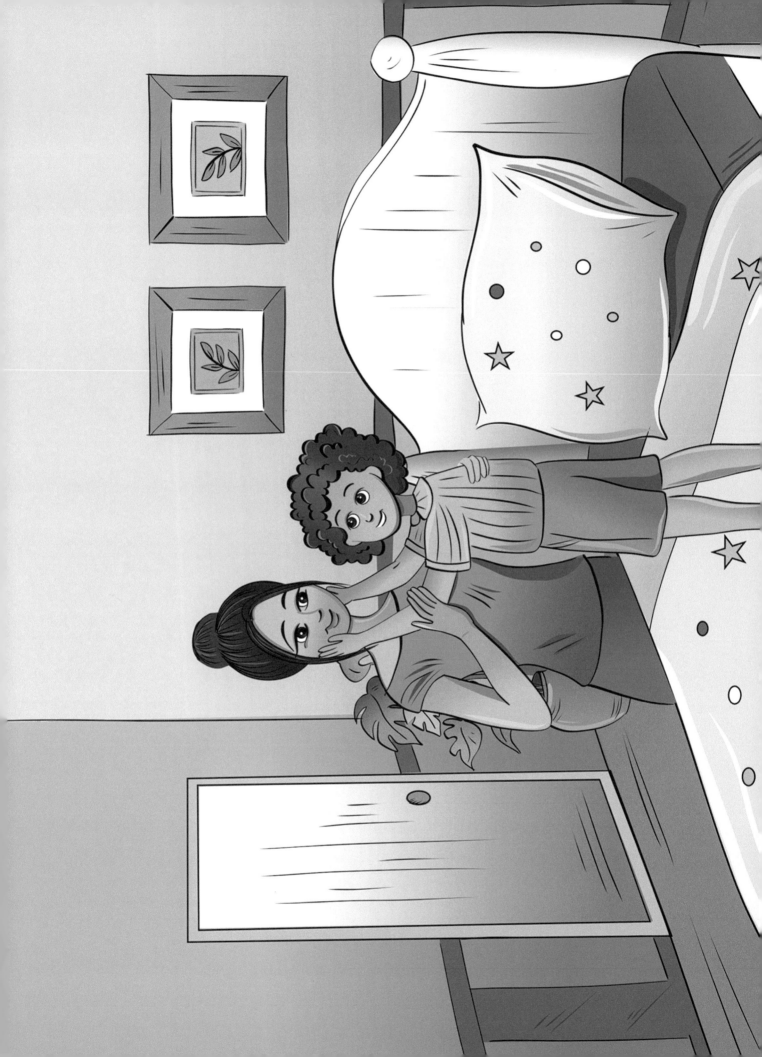

"WHAT!!!"

"What do we do? Where do we go?"

Mom said gently, "We will take you to Daddy's Barber – the one that you know."

"You mean that man in the window, who just stands and stares behind that big chair?"

"Oh Mommy! NO! I cannot go there! He makes me so scared!"

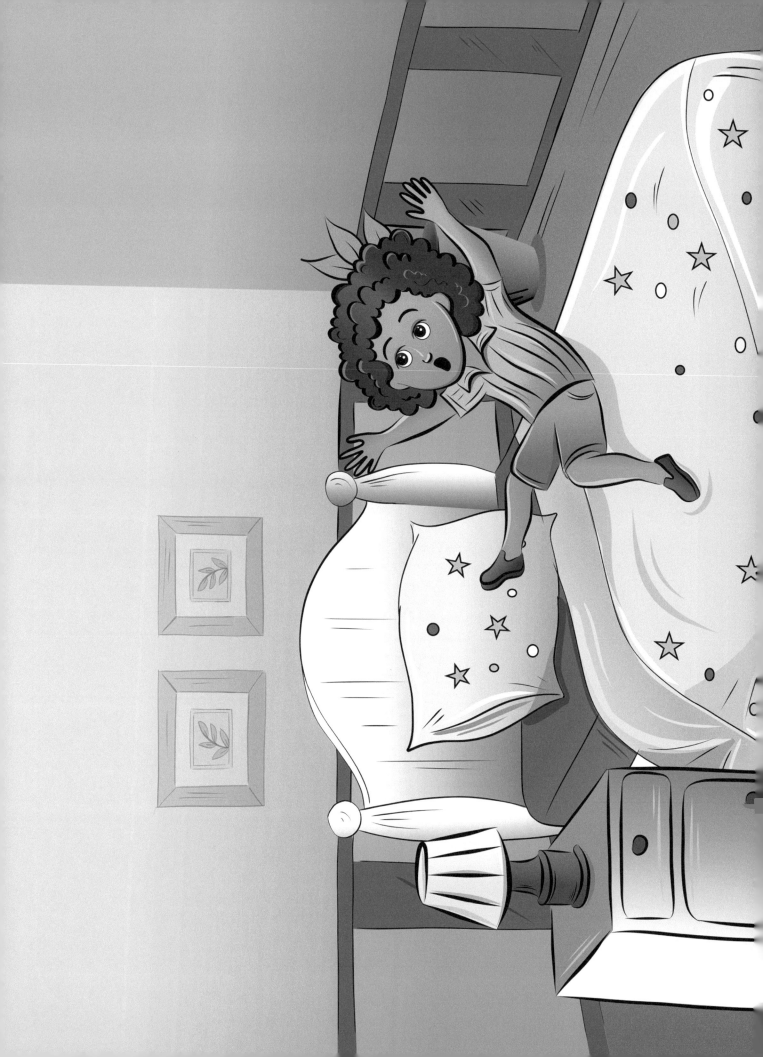

Mom smiled. "Don't you worry, it will be fine! Just wait until morning, we will go about nine."

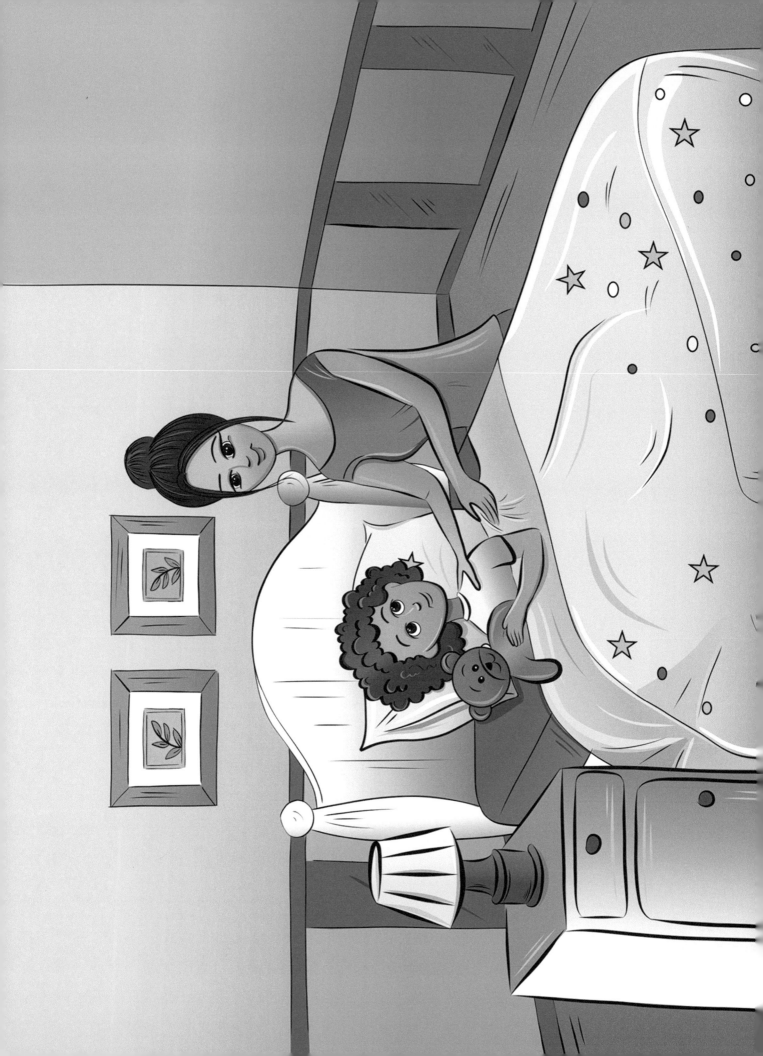

Believe it or not, I fell quickly to sleep......

And while dreaming my dreams,

Some new thoughts started to creep...

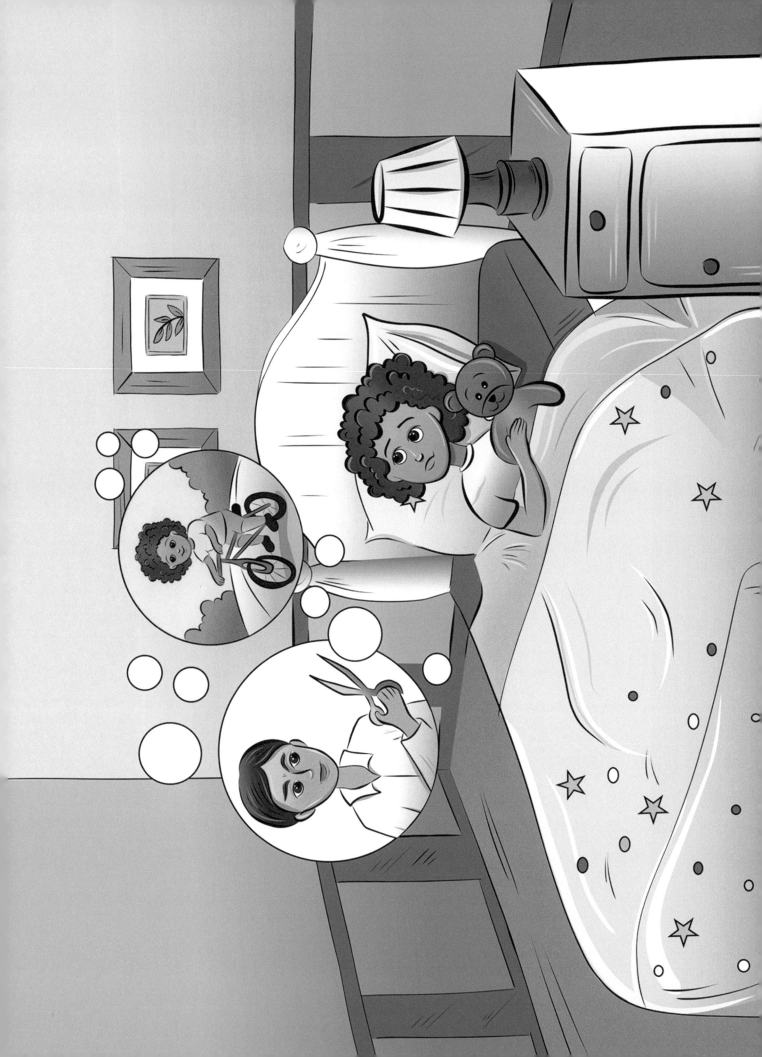

In the morning, I woke with a start when I heard my Mommy calling, "Wake up sweetheart!"

I called back, "I'm too sleepy today! I cannot wake up. I am too tired to play. I think I will just stay in my bed all day."

"Up we go Billy! Today's a big day! After breakfast you will have time to play, then we'll be on our way!"

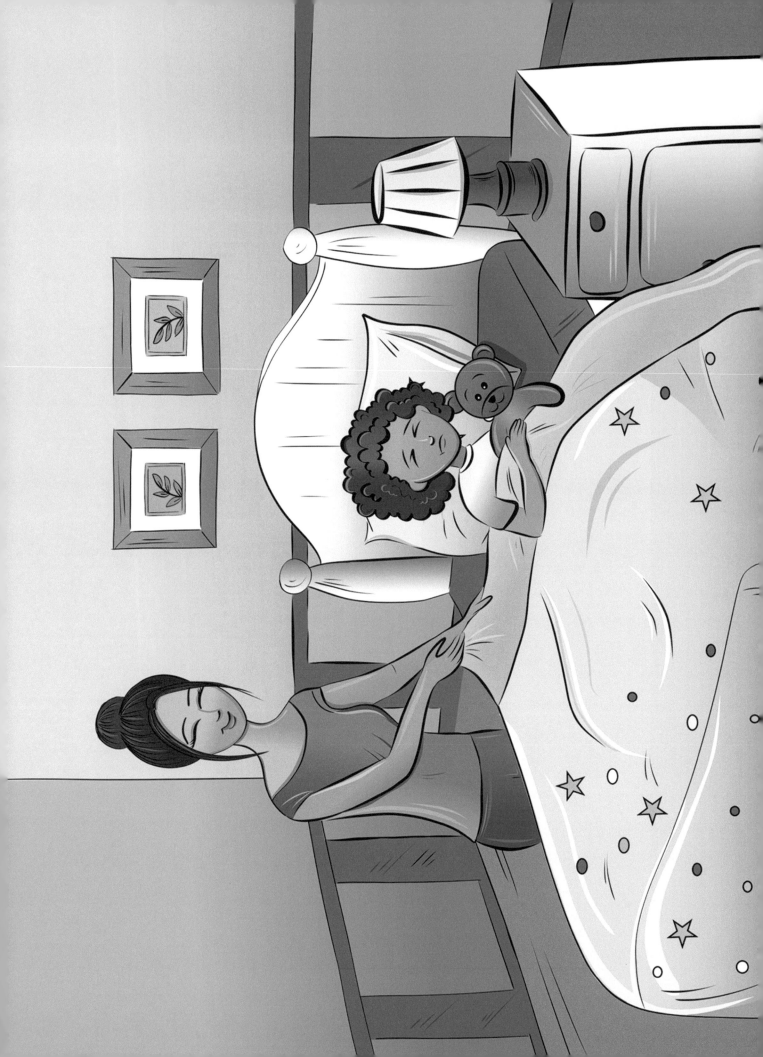

I ate breakfast and played and then the clock chimed.

Dad said, "Let's get ready.It's just about time."

We climbed in the car.

Pretty soon, we were there. I saw through the window:

The Barber. The Scissors. The Chair.

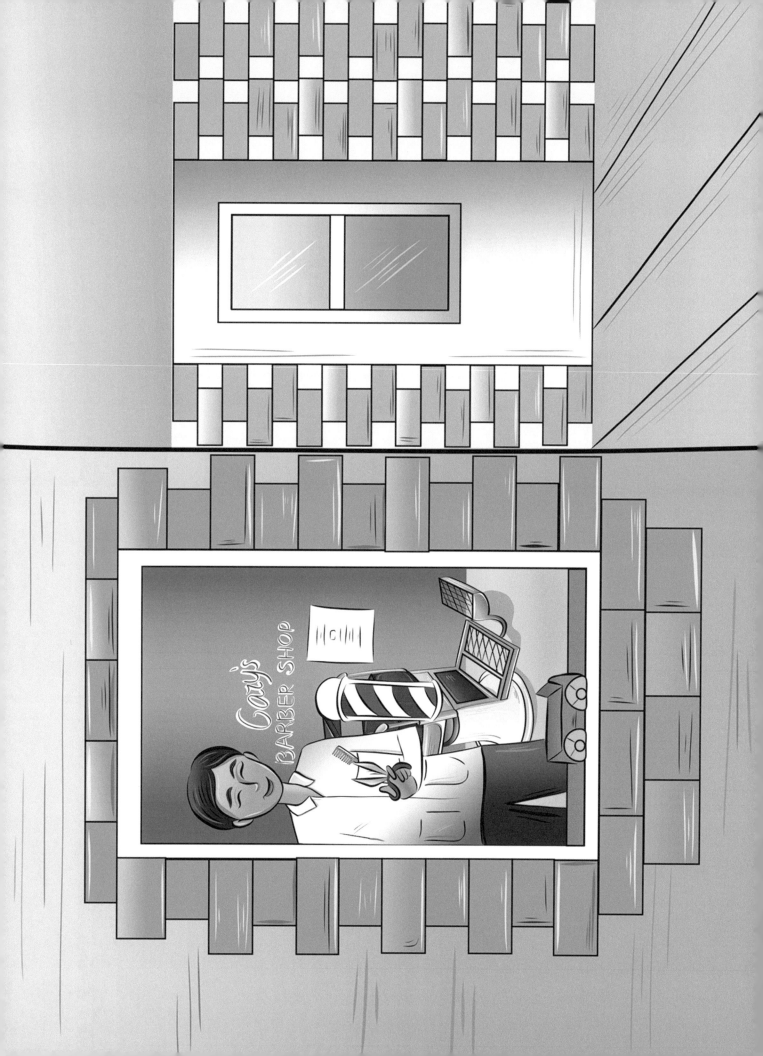

Daddy parked right in front and said, "Out you you go - He's waiting for you."

I hopped out of the car and walked to the door.

Then I panicked –

THIS WAS NOT WHAT I WANTED TO DO!

My Mom said, "Oh dear! Billy! Put your feet on the floor!"

Then Daddy picked me up - we went right through the door.

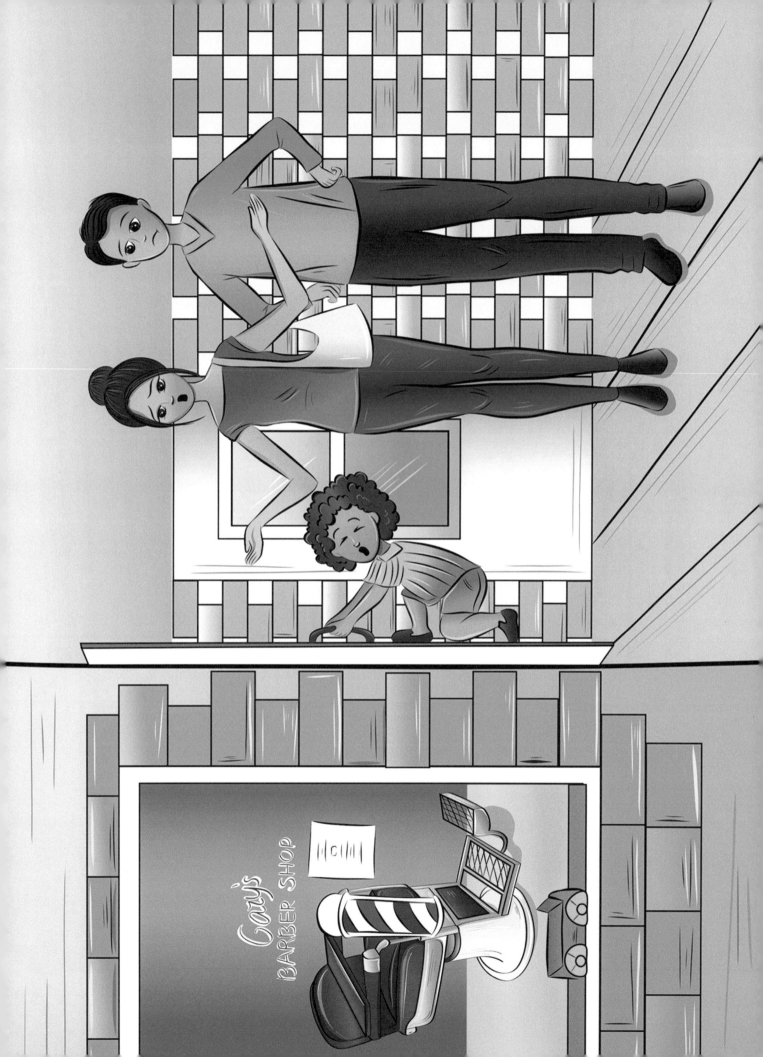

The Barber put a board across the arms of the chair.

He said to me, "Hi Billy! Up you hop there!"

I climbed up and sat down, then said "Wow! I'm up so high!"

He told me "That's so I can reach you, big guy."

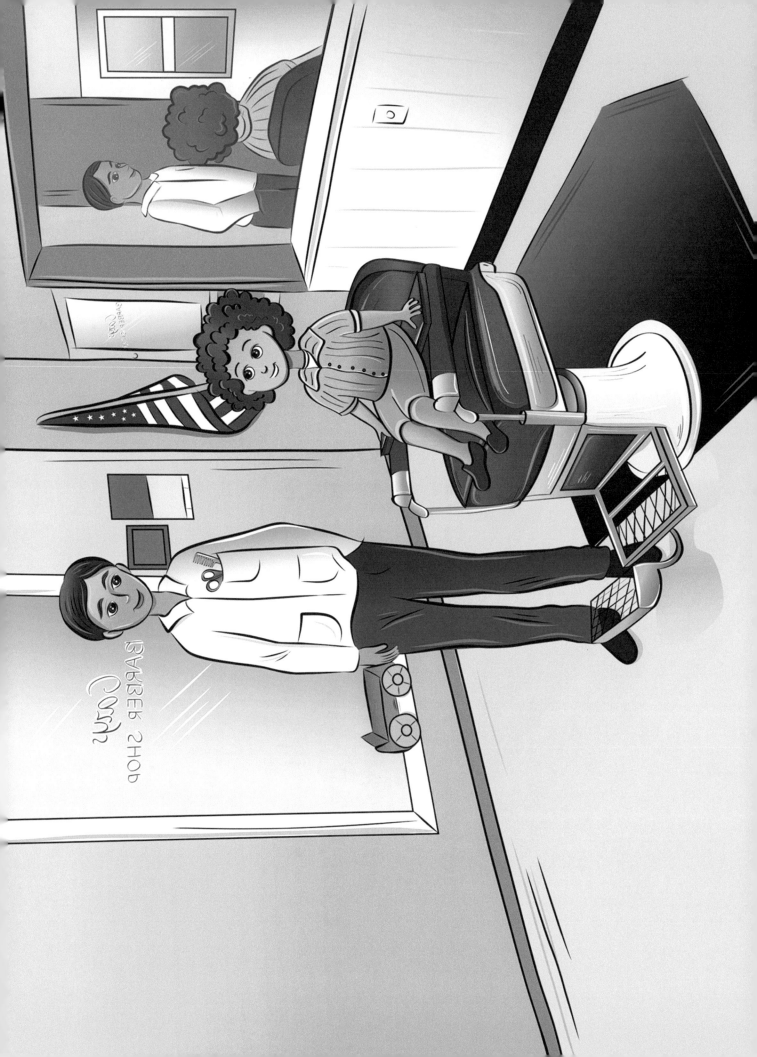

He told me, "I'll comb through your hair to get your tangles and all. Then, I'll snip off your curls, and down they will fall. When that is all done, I will straighten the line with the clippers. It will tickle your neck!"

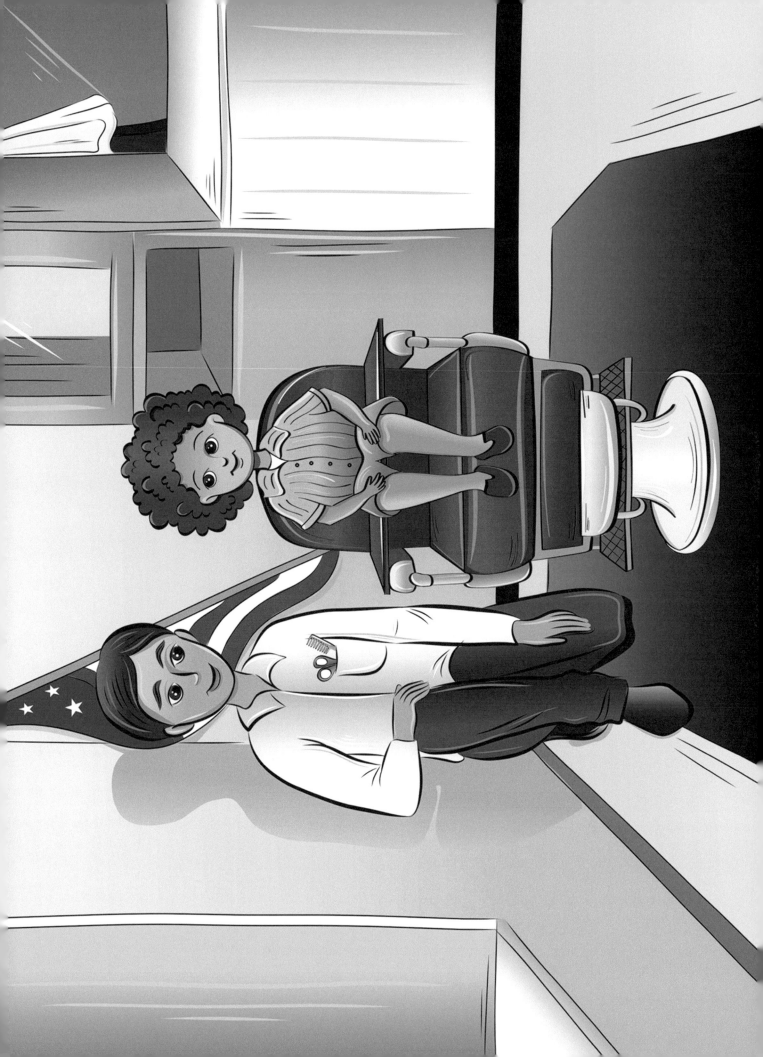

I closed my eyes tight. "Daddy, please stay nearby. Mommy, you too. Okay, Mr. Barber. Do what you have to do!"

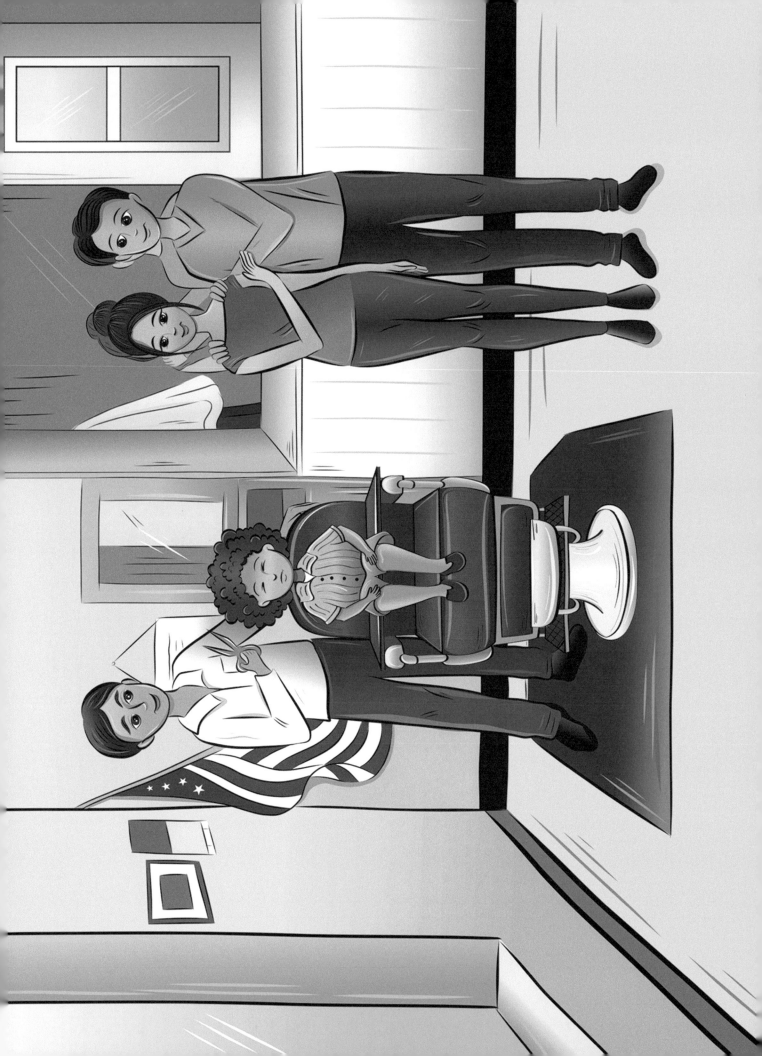

I felt the comb slide through my hair, tangles, and all.

I heard the scissors go snip, snip, snip! My curls start to fall.

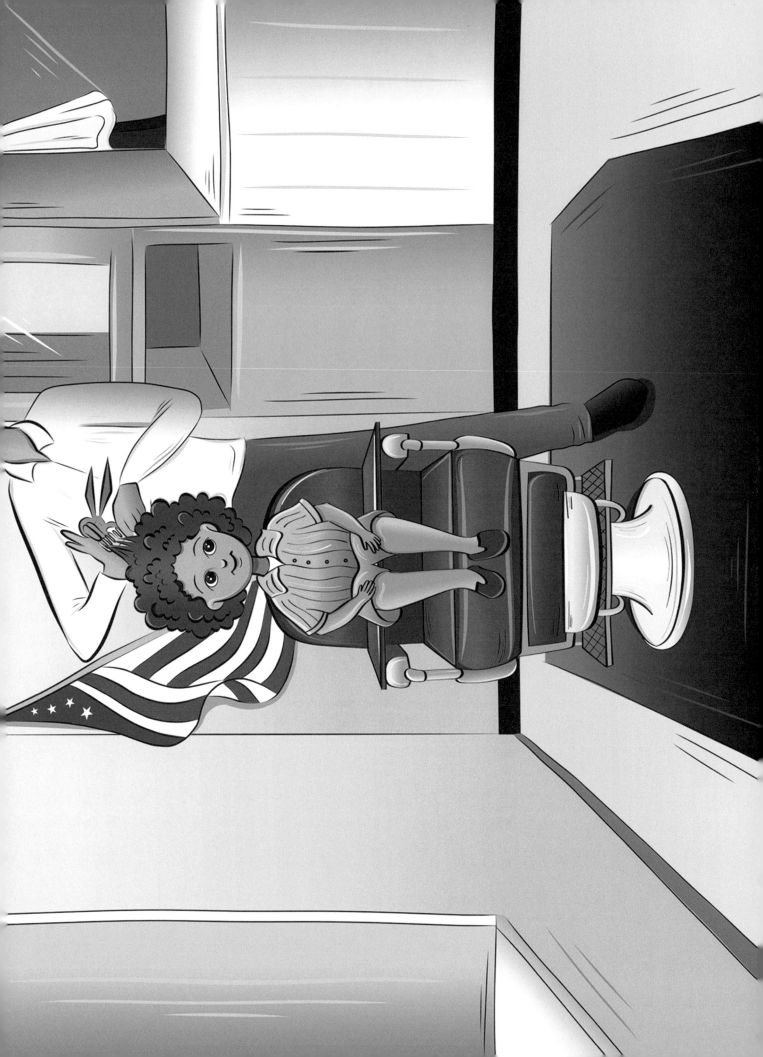

Mr. Barber said, "That's about it."

I was surprised. "It didn't hurt at all! Is it done?"

The Barber responded, "Almost. Bend your head down now."

I heard a loud buzzing and thought what now? I laughed cause the clippers tickled my neck!

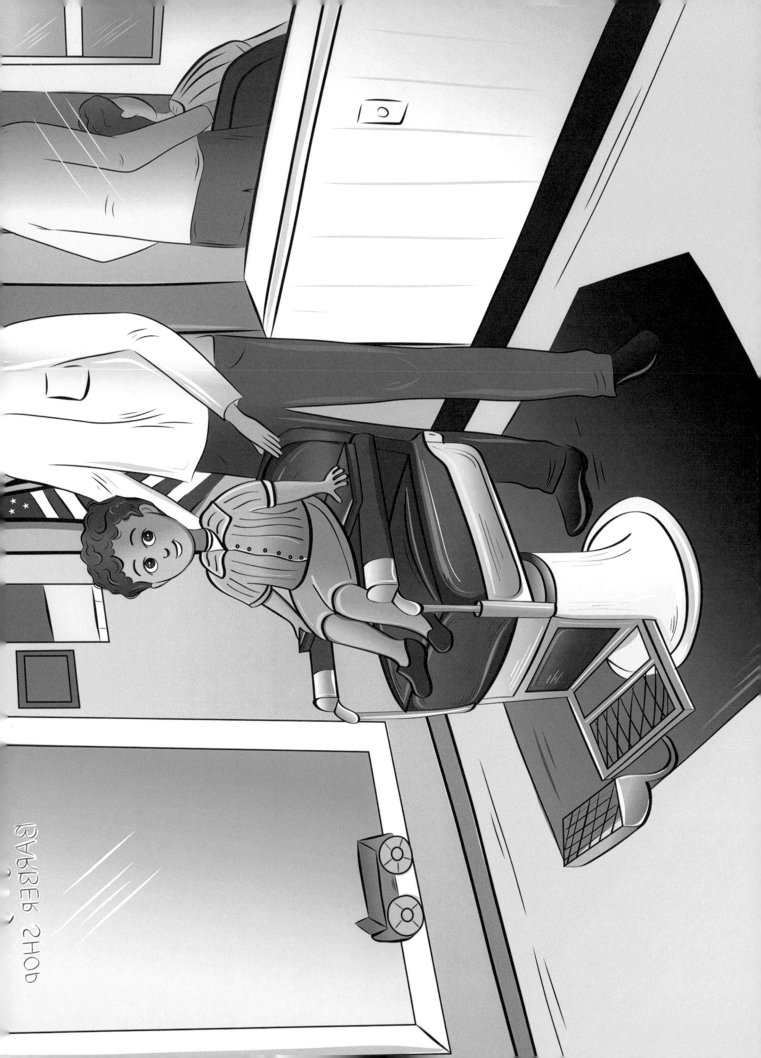

The Barber says, "You're all done. Look!"

I peeked with one eye, and then looked with two.

I could hardly believe that is all that it took.

My Daddy said, "Hey! You look handsome!"

And I said, "I do! I look like a big boy! My hair looks like new!"

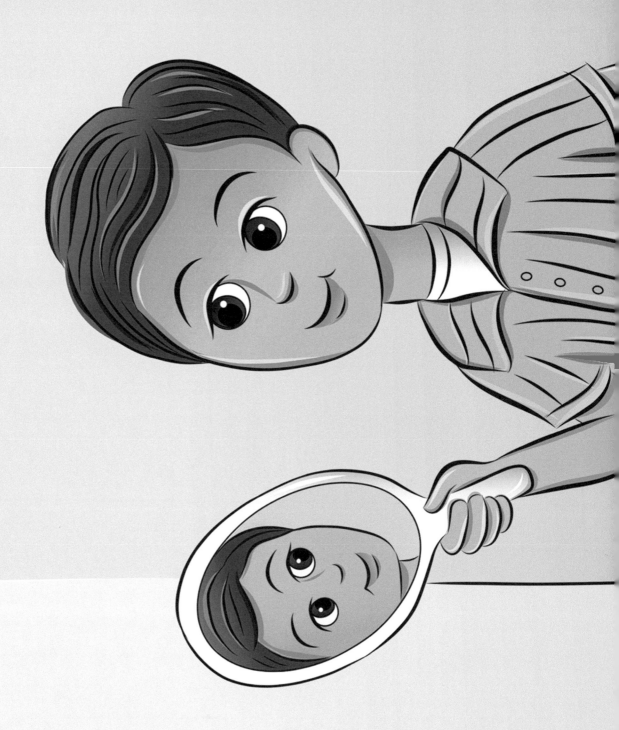

My Mommy and Daddy, and I smiled too.

Then Mom snapped a picture of my new hairdo!

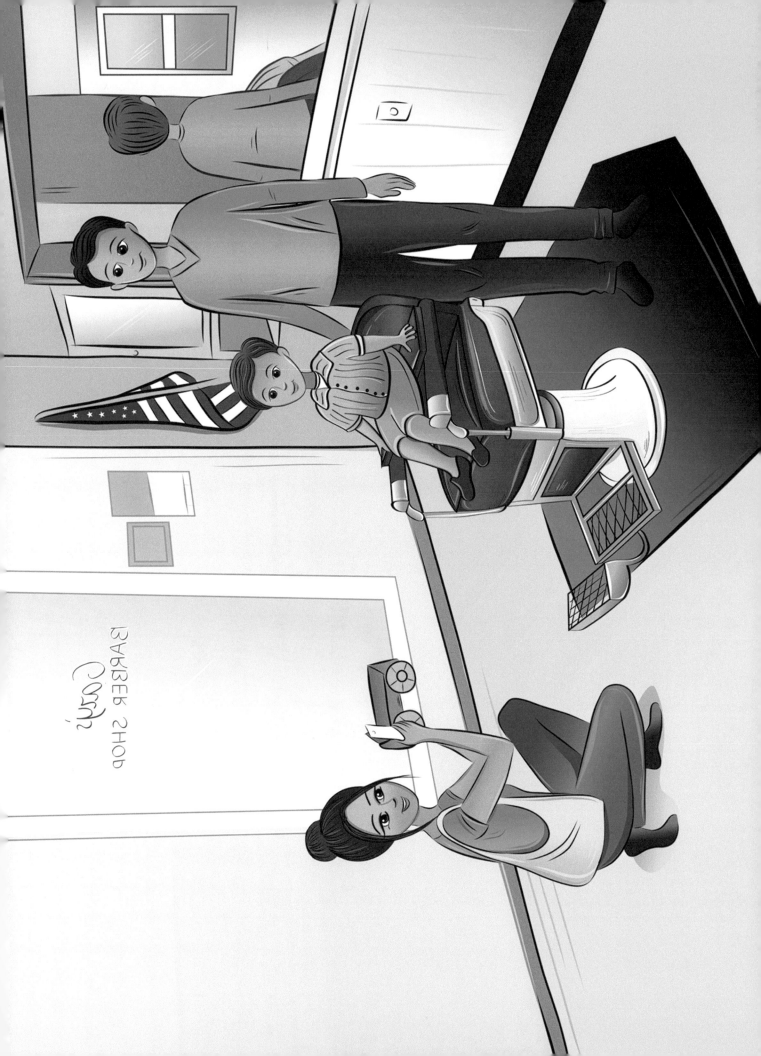

"Now there is one more thing we must do," the Barber said, "Come with me."

I said, "Wait! There's more?"

He took my hand, and we went next door.

"When you have your first haircut, we go to the candy store! You get a treat! You were such a good boy!"

I picked out some candy and one with a toy!

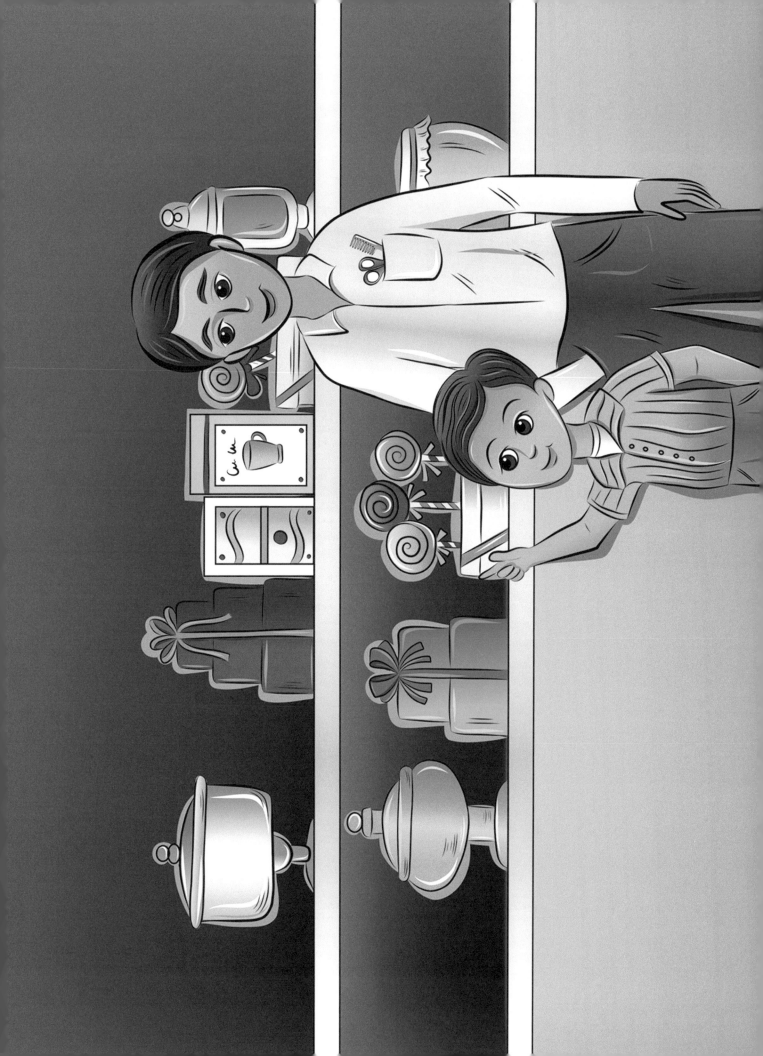

Back at the shop, I saw Mom bend down
to pick up a curl; in her eye was a tear.

I Said, "Oh, Mom, don't be sad! It was the bestime
I ever had! I'll tell all my friends
there is nothing to fear!"

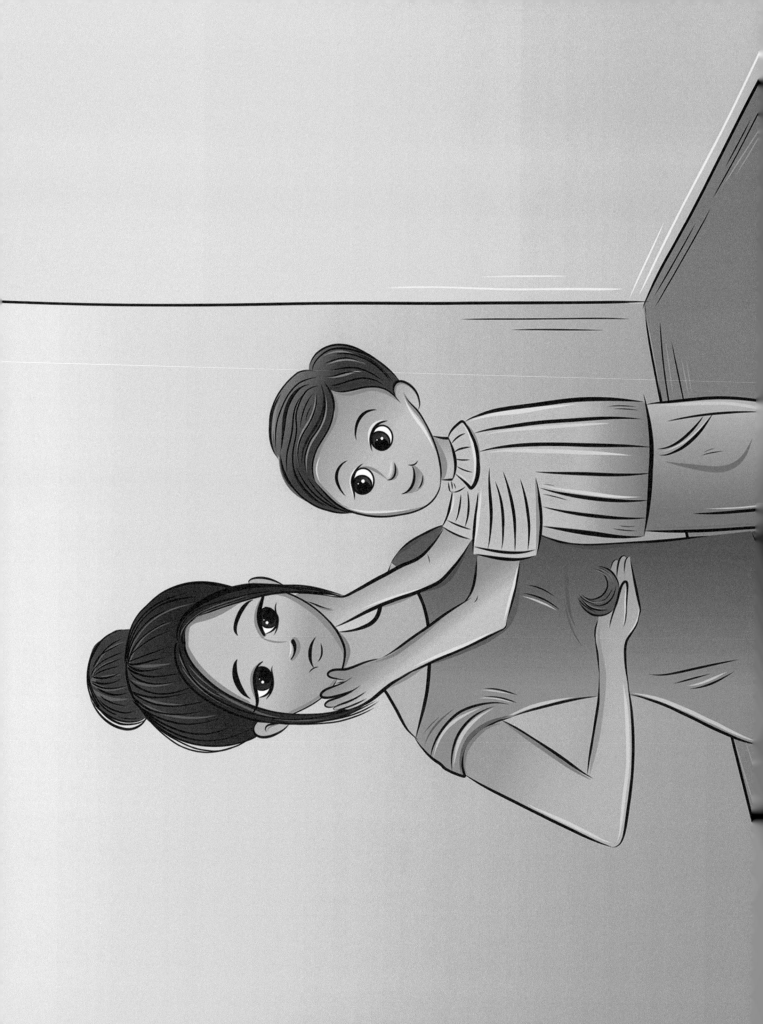

I like getting my haircut, I even got candy!

You were right; my haircut turned out just dandy!

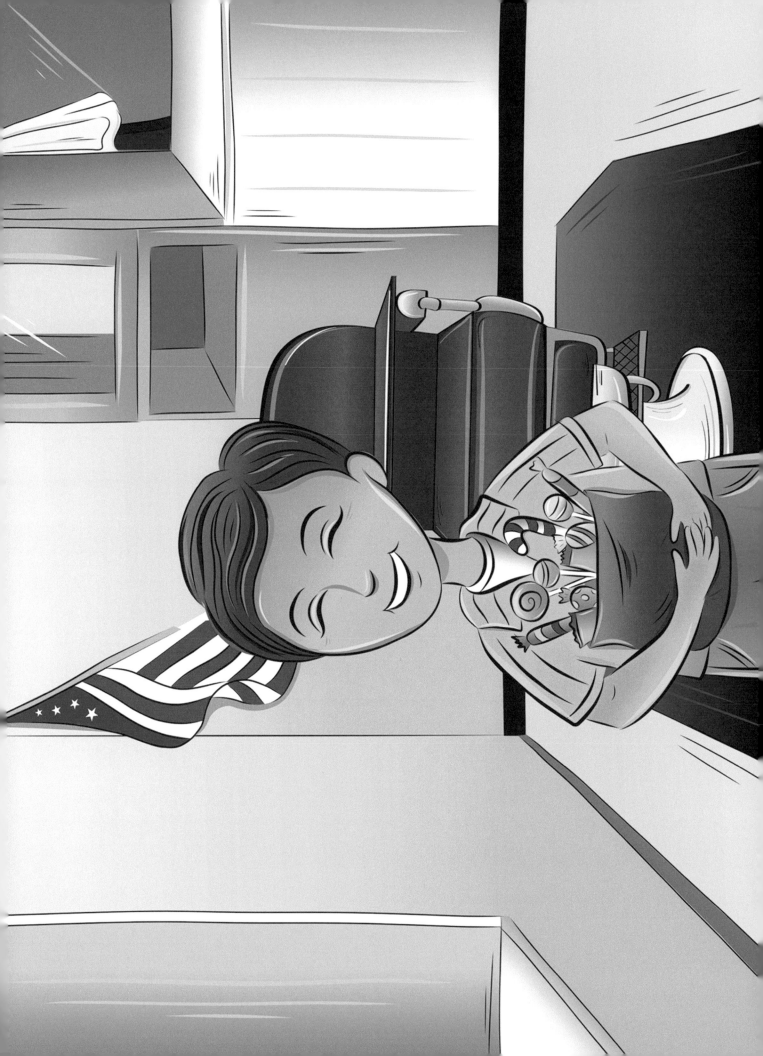

Printed in the United States
by Baker & Taylor Publisher Services